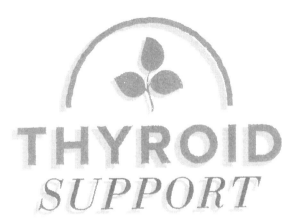

THYROID
SUPPORT

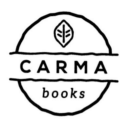

'A conscious approach to health & wellness'

carmabooks.com

*You are invited to to join our **Free Book Club** mailing list. Sign up via our website to receive **special offers** and **free for a limited time** Health & Wellness eBooks!*

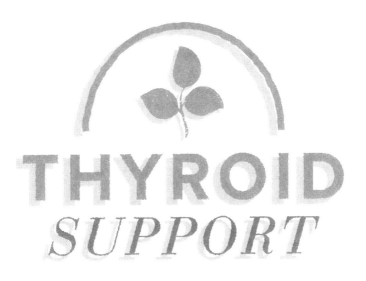

THYROID SUPPORT

20+ Herbal Remedies & Strategies to Banish Brain Fog, Boost Your Metabolism & Heal Your Underactive Thyroid Naturally

Carmen Reeves

Disclaimer

This book provides general information and extensive research regarding health and related subjects. The information provided in this book, and in any linked materials is for informational purposes only, and is not intended to be construed as medical advice. Speak with your physician or other healthcare professional before taking any nutritional or herbal supplements. There are no 'typical' results from the information provided - as individuals differ, the results will differ. Before considering any guidance from this book, please ensure you do not have any underlying health conditions which may interfere with the suggested healing methods. If the reader or any other person has a medical concern or pre-existing condition, he or she should consult with an appropriately licensed physician or healthcare professional. Never disregard professional medical advice or delay in seeking it because of something you have read in this book or in any linked materials. The reader assumes the risk and full responsibility for all actions, and the author or publisher will not be held liable for any loss or damage that may result from the information presented in this publication.

Carma Books
carmabooks.com

hello@carmabooks.com

CONTENTS

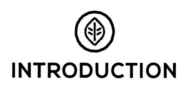

INTRODUCTION

I deeply thank you and congratulate you on your purchase of my latest publication—*Thyroid Support: 20+ Herbal Remedies & Strategies to Banish Brain Fog, Boost Your Metabolism & Heal Your Underactive Thyroid Naturally.* I hope that my own personal experience, research, and acquaintanceship with close friends, family, and other sufferers of hypothyroid dysfunction will be of benefit to you, the reader!

But I don't just hope—I know for a fact that this book will be of help to you. No doubt you have found this book because you are trying to find better understanding of thyroid issues, and to start your own journey into better self-knowledge, empowerment, and confidence in handling the matter. Before stepping into the complex and misunderstood world of thyroid health, I was very much in those same shoes.

The First Step is the Hardest... Then it Gets Easier

Every path can have a difficult beginning. Maybe you don't know much on the subject of thyroid issues at all, or you have a friend, family member, or patient who is undergoing struggles that have caused you to reach out for further education.

Perhaps you are even experiencing the telltale signs

of hypothyroid issues yourself. **Depression, brain fog, and fatigue—classic symptoms of a hypo-thyroid—overshadow the wellness and energy you or loved ones desire and miss so much, and it can be incredibly hard to take that first step towards finding some answers,** especially when you are bogged down with the symptoms of an underactive thyroid.

In fact, so many people don't even take that first step. The symptoms of hypothyroidism itself are so discouraging, dogging you at every turn, that they make the journey towards healing seem all the harder; while reaching out to doctors and health professionals can yield only more questions than answers, and possibly even worsened thyroid health, in some cases.

Some people don't even take that first step because they have no idea these symptoms can be connected to a disorder. Even the American Thyroid Association states that close to **60% of those with thyroid conditions are completely unaware that they have a thyroid problem**.

This is the very purpose behind me writing this book. Again, I congratulate you on taking that first step, which is always the hardest. But from here on out, with the information you find here, it *will* get easier!

My Own Story with Hypothyroid

Many, many years ago, a close friend and teacher/mentor of mine herself became a sufferer of thyroid issues. This began my own journey into understanding the thyroid, a first step that was much too difficult for my dear teacher to make herself.

What was most alarming and scary was that she was a master, expert, and professional in the health industry herself. She was the figure who mentored me and taught me all that she knew. But there she was: fatigued, foggy and discouraged, with too many responsibilities and too little energy to find answers herself.

She was gaining weight, even starting to lose some of her hair, and developing some hard-to-diagnose digestive disorders. Arthritis-like symptoms set in as well, giving her body aches and pains. But the scariest moment was when she experienced almost complete kidney shut down, for which she had to be rushed to the hospital.

With her unable to take the reins, I did what I could to help her. I researched publications, studies, and online journals. I liaised with health professionals who were more adept and eyeful of thyroid problems, and avoided doctors who had never handled it nor researched it. I also got involved in organizations and gatherings centered around the subject of thyroid issues, to learn and experience more.

Today, my dear friend and teacher manages her underactive thyroid on her own: through diet, herbs, and deeply-instilled lifestyle changes, with less dependence and support on any modern medications. **This knowledge that she and I cobbled together, through our experiences and research, is very much the**

foundation for the contents of this book—and you are now welcome and able to access that yourself!

There is simply no measuring how much all that knowledge, data, and wisdom has helped me gain a perspective on so many dimensions of my health and others' health, all of which I have carefully collected and experienced over the years.

But not just concerning the thyroid alone: practically *ALL* aspects of health and wellness, too. In learning more about hypothyroidism, how it works, and even healing it naturally, I have become more equipped against a wide variety of health issues than I could have ever imagined.

Hypothyroidism: Silent and Misunderstood

Beyond my personal experiences, why is hypothyroidism a big deal? Firstly, it is much more widespread among the population than some might think, and growing fast as a diagnosed illness. But it can also be incredibly hard to pinpoint and diagnose certain hypothyroid disorders, in some cases.

Even though there are very specific methods of detecting and diagnosing them, various thyroid problems can be so subtle or imperceptible that they are easily overlooked by health practitioners. Worse, those who are suffering from hypothyroid problems may not even realize it until much further down the road, when problems are already deep and have taken hold.

Statistics gathered by the American Thyroid Association (ATA) allege that **somewhere over 20 million Americans suffer from some type of thyroid disease**. Again, nearly 2/3 of these sufferers have no idea that they have a thyroid problem—up to 60%. This is why underactive thyroid ranks among ailments that seem like "silent killers"—its onset can be gradual, but the consequences and implications are drastic.

Don't worry: thyroid problems are not directly fatal in most cases! But thyroid dysfunction can have a hand in other greater diseases and illnesses that develop in the body, such as they did with my teacher and friend.

If you, as you are reading this, are suspecting that you could be having some thyroid struggles—it is important that you follow those instincts and address them sooner than later. **In spite of what any doctor will tell you: yes, it *IS* important.**

An untreated thyroid condition could possibly give way to other health complications, both big and small. More commonly, hypothyroid is suspected of contributing to some of the wider population's struggles with malaise, fatigue, depression, weight gain, digestive disorders, and even heart disease. Do any of these symptoms seem familiar among yourself or your loved ones?

This is exactly why knowledge is the most powerful thing in handling an underactive thyroid; not just any knowledge, but the truest, deepest knowledge possible from multiple perspectives: both conventional and alternative.

Mysterious Causes, with Evidence for Treatment

Layered with hypothyroidism's quiet and sometimes unnoticed onset, the actual causes of the problem itself are also not very transparent, and hard to pinpoint. The American Thyroid Association and scientific study state that thyroid issue causes are mostly unknown, for now.

This makes for a very difficult approach: for a functioning gland with far-reaching but complex influences on the body, the reasons for it developing a disorder are also intricate, and sometimes impossible to trace to any one trigger or cause.

Recent studies do elucidate some very strong evidence and possible pathways for treatment, however. **Hypothyroidism correlates to immunity, genetics, metabolism, hormone health, cellular function, nutritional, and digestive health, among many others.** Since it is clearly bound in influence on all organ systems of the body, then it can be easily said that many bodily functions in turn have their impact on the thyroid.

Science also demonstrates a marked relation of thyroid hormone production to both gut health/digestion processes, as well as unnatural levels of harmful, chronic inflammation. These two targets for thyroid health will be discussed thoroughly in the following pages, but you can also explore the topics in my other two books: *Healthy Gut Solution* and *Natural Anti-Inflammatory Remedies.*

Even for me the research and learning is not over! While

there is still a "shroud of mystery" around thyroid causes, nevertheless I can attest to the knowledge and experiences I myself compiled and practiced while helping my dear teacher, and educating others. Yet there is still so much to learn and research, and I can attest to that as well.

For a journey into all topics related to thyroid health, however, please read on. The pages ahead contain my experiences and research with underactive thyroid, revealing my own personal observations and methods of success. I have seen these tips and knowledge sprout and grow successfully among friends, family, and other sufferers of this overlooked, misunderstood health issue. Let this be your road map in navigating the complex world of hypothyroidism, and a great way also for you to spread some amazing knowledge and education. For our next and first chapter, a great place to start on understanding thyroid matters begins with the simple question: ***"What is the thyroid, and what does it do?"***

CHAPTER 1

What is the thyroid, and how does it work?

You might hear quite a bit about the thyroid these days. But a lot of even the most health-savvy people might not know exactly what the thyroid does!

It is an admittedly small part of anatomy, filed under the Endocrine System dealing with metabolism, proteins, and hormones. In fact, the **Endocrine System** itself is not talked about too much in popular physiology—being overshadowed by others such as the Nervous, Muscular, or Respiratory Systems, for example.

This does not make this vital system any less important or irrelevant—and might be one of the reasons why it is so overlooked in mainstream health. The Endocrine System governs the function and role of glands in the body, and there are many different glands in all, each designed to govern and mediate various roles. Bodily actions that glands have a hand in include **sexual function, sleep, natural tissue growth,** and even our **mood and energy levels**.

Glands can produce, emit, and secrete various hormones, proteins, and neuro-transmitters that are sent throughout the bloodstream. These, in a way, communicate "messages" and specific operations to tissues in the body to regulate, increase, or decrease certain processes.

What are some other glands and h**
you might have heard about, besi**
thyroid? Well, one of the most commonly discussed is the **Pituitary Gland** that governs sex hormones like estrogen, progestin and testosterone.

There is also the **Adrenal Gland**, master of energy and stress levels, which produces adrenaline and cortisone. You can read all about Adrenal Gland health in another one of my publications: *Adrenal Fatigue: Cure it Naturally.*

In the pages ahead, we will take a close examination of the thyroid gland: where it is located, and even its roles connected to other major bodily systems. How it functions will also be explored next, with some preview on how dysfunction can (and does) happen.

The Thyroid Gland

Located in the neck, the thyroid is often referred to as "butterfly shaped," wrapped neatly around the trachea or "windpipe." You can even feel the thyroid with your hand: try touching the base of your neck just above your clavicle, and right below the "Adam's Apple." (Yes... even in women!)

While other glands might secrete and transmit hormones that regulate sexual function or digestion, **the thyroid specializes in hormones that govern heart rate,**

od pressure, body temperature, energy use from food, and metabolism.

What's important to note, however, is that these processes are baseline to practically every other function in the body. Hormones released by the thyroid can interact and have an influence on every single human cell, as a matter of fact.

How does it work? The thyroid first receives messages from the **hypothalamus** and **anterior pituitary gland** in the brain, which then stimulate it to secrete and broadcast its own set of hormones to yet more systems and other glands in the body. The hypothalamus can be thought of almost like a *"pressure gauge,"* a highly centrifugal gland that scans aspects of health like nutrition, hormones, temperature, and other important contents in the blood.

With what information the hypothalamus detects, the pituitary acts upon. It sends hormones to the thyroid, triggering a chain-reaction for the thyroid itself to then take action and balance the body in reaction to the information perceived by the hypothalamus, so the body maintains wellness, health and harmony.

The hormone sent from the pituitary to the thyroid is commonly called **TSH**, or **Thyroid Stimulating Hormone**.

TSH – Thyroid Stimulating Hormone

This hormone stimulates the thyroid to work in one way or another, but always for the purpose of maintaining balance in the body's metabolism, blood pressure, and energy use functions. It either **increases** the levels of hormones the thyroid produces, or it decreases them, all depending on what the hypothalamus detects in the bloodstream.

For example: if the body experiences increased activity or colder temperatures, more TSH will be released to boost body temperature and improve the production of heat from food (calories), thus creating more energy to be used.

If the opposite happens—high temperatures, or less activity, for example—metabolism is slowed under the thyroid, with less TSH being released to encourage reserved energy usage and maintain healthy homeo-stasis.

With an active thyroid, you have more energy; with an underactive thyroid, you could feel fatigued or slowed down.

Basically, TSH is the hormone that regulates the thyroid itself from the "control room" of the hypothalamus/ pituitary gland. When there's more TSH, the thyroid begins producing more if its own particular hormones that then mediate and interact with all cellular function in the body.

The names of the thyroid's proper hormones are T3 and T4, or **triidothyrinine** and **thyroxine** respectively.

T3 – Triidothyrinine, the Thyroid "Powerhouse"

Considered one of the key, "target" hormones to evaluate in thyroid health, T3 is produced when TSH reaches the thyroid, initiating a cocktail of bio-chemistry. Enzymes and proteins like thyroglobulin and thyroid peroxidase combine in a medley with iodine pulled from blood-stream nutrients: and presto, T3 (and its companion, T4) are created.

Between T3 and T4, T3 is the most active—endo-crinologists state that it can be anywhere from 4 to 10 times more influential than T4 as a thyroid hormone, furthering positive bodily function. However, during the TSH-stimulation process, only about 7% of the hormones created are T3, while the remaining 93% are mostly the less-effective T4.

This is why T3 is not only considered the "powerhouse" thyroid hormone, but the best one to target for increasing thyroid health. Its numbers are the most likely to dwindle, leading way to diminished thyroid function, even hypothyroidism.

It must be understood, however, that while the body doesn't naturally and directly produce great amounts of healthy T3, it can boost its levels by other means. One of the main ways for it to do so is by **converting T4 into T3, transforming thyroxine into triiodothyronine**—but this depends on the health and function of various other bodily systems as part of the bigger picture.

T4 – Thryoxine, the Thyroid "Proliferator"

"Prolific" means to be plentiful and populous, and that is certainly what T4 is: a "proliferator," responsible and capable of increasing (or, decreasing) needed thyroid levels, by acting almost like the body's major "reserves." T4 is found in very large amounts circulating throughout the body and bloodstream, and has some small effect on calibrating certain energy functions critical to the thyroid's purpose. **One of its primary callings, however, is its readiness to be transformed from T4 into T3 when need be.**

60% of all T4 circulates to the liver, in order to be converted into needed T3. Another 20% becomes available to the gut for further T3 production and use and is processed in the intestine. This strongly links digestive health to thyroid health, it is true, and we will be delving into the importance of the thyroid/gut connection later in this book.

Consequentially, T4 amounts are just as important as T3 ones, but in a different way and for different processes. It may seem with all this description that there appears to be abundant levels of thyroid levels coursing through the blood, ready and able to regulate all cellular and systemic function when need be.

But one must realize that a great extent of T4 and T3 can become "bound up" by other proteins and enzymes in the blood, making them "unusable" as thyroid hormones needed by the anatomical processes that require them. **In fact, only .03% of T4 produced by the thyroid is accessible in the bloodstream, coupled with .3% of produced T3!**

This is exactly why thyroid levels are so important to observe and keep track of in the bigger picture of total health. If overlooked, and allowed to dip into unhealthy levels—then you start experiencing the tiredness, fatigue, brain fog, and other symptoms of a hypothyroid.

We'll take a closer look at that in one of the chapters ahead: *"What leads to an unhappy, underactive thyroid?"* But since we have covered the basic thyroid actions and purposes for now, let's gain a better understanding of this major gland's functions when healthy, allowing us better learning of its role in the body.

This leads us to our next chapter: ***"Why is the thyroid vital to health and vibrancy?"***

CHAPTER 2

Why is the thyroid vital to health and vibrancy?

In the previous chapter, we took a simple but thorough look at how the thyroid functions. Levels of its principal hormones—T3 and T4—are the thin dividing line between thyroid health, and thyroid dysfunction. In this chapter, we'll study how these levels affect the body: particularly when they are working correctly, doing all they should do, and promoting optimal health in organs elsewhere in human anatomy.

If there was a way to perfectly encapsulate and define thyroid's role in the body—what would it be? This is an excellent question, and its answer can help you—the reader—get to the very bottom of thyroid understanding and, even better, its management!

Think of your thyroid like the "accelerator" in your car. Your body needs fuel, just like your car does. The thyroid regulates how your body uses this fuel, and also where it goes in the body where it's needed the most, especially in terms of energy consumption and cellular activity. Like the gas pedal in your car, it can decide to burn more energy, or slow it down when less activity is needed.

Even further, the thyroid can be a lot like the "catalytic converter" in a vehicle. Over time, when this car part stops working so well, it can effect fuel efficiency—burning up or misusing way too much fuel just to maintain some of the simplest bodily processes. A car might have a very hard time getting started and maintaining speed if a catalytic converter problem is the case, just like someone has issues with tiredness, fatigue, and concentration with an underactive thyroid.

It can be said that the thyroid is like your "fuel efficiency." You want the very best mileage that your body can possibly get, and having a hypothyroid problem could drop your mileage and energy levels. In anatomy and physiology, the process of bodily fuel efficiency is called **"metabolism."**

Metabolism

When all is well with the thyroid, this means that metabolism is in excellent working condition. You are getting all the optimal distance and mileage your body should be getting, on the adequate fuel and foods your body requires. You're full of energy, alertness, and a zest for life!

Metabolism defines the "speed" at which cells in the body use up energy from food or nutrients, and the thyroid's principal hormones—T3 and T4—have the final say in this. Passing through the bloodstream, they interact with every cell throughout your body, whether that be a cell in your brain, in your intestine, or in your pinky toe (it doesn't matter!).

Wherever T3 or T4 mediates with a cell, they encourage a faster rate of metabolism. That being: faster energy consumption, energy usage, fat burning, and heat production, to be specific. Cells begin to use more energy, and bodily processes accelerate. **Energy needs and nutrient levels are all aspects of the body that the hypothalamus keeps tabs on, like we discussed in the previous chapter, but they are played out through the thyroid to make sure energy usage and processing is "just right."**

It's the hypothalamus that tracks and encourages those wonderful energy levels and concentration we all hope for and work towards for good health!

When it is determined that the body doesn't need to burn, create, or process as much energy, then the hypothalamus withholds TSH, which then withholds T3 and T4 from creation in the thyroid. It's only when the hypothalamus sees needs for more energy, that these are increased once more through this endocrine chain reaction between the pituitary and thyroid glands—and metabolism is sped up all over again!

For one reason or another, when the thyroid fails to act upon what the hypothalamus detects, that's when our bodies struggle with energy.

Micro- and Macro-nutrient Uses

These are related to metabolism as well, though they are considered somewhat more "specialized" functions that aren't only linked to energy usage. T3 and T4 do play primary roles in the "burning" of nutrients like fuel, but they also delegate them toward other uses, like new tissue growth or maintenance.

Macronutrients like fats, proteins, and glucose (sugars) are responsible for a lot of energy, but they are also used for energy storage and bodily growth. Thyroid hormones toggle the switch controlling the burning of these macronutrients in cells for energy, but are also instrumental to taking them in and allocating them to either grow or support tissues in the body. One place where they are absolutely integral is the **brain** for healthy mental processes, as well as helping make new proteins for all sorts of developing tissues that need them.

Through the metabolizing of proteins and sugars as well, the thyroid also facilitates trigger for fat burning and storage—but it also participates in the processing of **calcium, magnesium and phosphorus**, very vital nutrients in the body.

For these micronutrients, this is actually connected to separate actions of the **parathyroid glands**, smaller thyroids found in and on the larger thyroid gland, which regulate the levels of these minerals in the blood.

Their use towards bone/muscle/organ health, and finally, output and excretion in urine, is controlled somewhat by these glands— making the thyroid and parathyroid all very important aspects of not just energy usage, but nutrient usage for the strength of the body, to boot. **After all: nutrients themselves are our**

literal fuels for energy!

Connection to All Bodily Functions and Organs

What makes the thyroid truly remarkable is its processing and allocation of micro- and macro-nutrients, which unarguably hold sway over all of human physiology. What organ, muscle, bone, or brain cell in the body could truly get away scot-free without the proper usage of fat, blood glucose, protein, calcium and magnesium?

As a result, the thyroid is a "gatekeeper" to health in all of our systems, whether it be the Skeletal, the Vascular, the Nervous, or even the Reproductive. It helps the body create and contribute proper building blocks for practically every possible organ and tissue, out of the most commonly used and necessary nutrients found in the human diet!

As a result, the thyroid is not just about our mileage, fuel, and energy overall. It governs the function and energy of every singular, separate, or inter-connected organ in our bodies!

Even further, however, the thyroid can have a direct, unique influence on us physically: one that side-steps just basic metabolism. For the Vascular system, it correlates to heightened heart beat and cardiac output, for example. For the Respiratory, it increases and supports our breathing, which then helps oxygen flow through our bloodstream to where it is needed.

Thyroid hormone levels can also "rev up" the Nervous System, creating more awareness, mental focus, and alertness by increasing sympathetic response. Finally, perfect thyroid balance contributes to uterine health in women, which then has a hand in strong fertility and reproduction. As you can see, the thyroid connects itself to much of the body!

For such a small gland, the thyroid should not be underestimated. When levels of T3 and T4 are at a healthy amount, all organs, systems, and their functions run smoothly. We have boundless levels of energy and vitality to go throughout our day, and meet with life's many challenges: stress, school, work and family.

The hypothalamus, found in our brain and working like the body's "pressure gauge", stays aware at all times of our current energy levels—by checking the bloodstream and the levels of thyroid hormones flowing there. At least, that is how the process is supposed to work, when all is well.

Thyroid T3 and T4 released from triggers in the hypo-thalamus then tell the body exactly what to do with what inputs the hypothalamus senses: such as stimuli, temperature, nutrients, and other factors. **But what happens if something goes wrong?**

For one reason or another, the thyroid sometimes releases T3 and T4 levels that are different and wrong in comparison to what the body needs to regulate and have energy. When this happens over a long period of time, a thyroid issue develops. **Modern science**

maintains that a predominant cause for this is mostly uncertain, but there are a number of culprits suspected that can give rise to thyroid dysfunction, according to mounting research.

Truthfully, the contributors to hypothyroid disorders can be numerous and complex, some of them even inter-connected in mysterious ways. Furthermore, modern medicine has found only few, incomplete methods to fully trace the onset of hypothyroidism to any one source.

Some methods work, and some methods don't—as tracking the proper hormones working the thyroid gland requires complete understanding, which some mainstream practitioners simply aren't trained or schooled in.

In the next chapter, we will get into the other side of thyroid function—in contrast to how this major gland should work when all is well, **we will next study what factors can lead to an unhealthy, underactive thyroid.**

CHAPTER 3

What leads to an unhappy, underactive thyroid?

When all is well with the thyroid, we use energy just as we should. We might even have tons of it! We can get all the possible mileage out of our bodies, if not more, if we make thyroid health a priority—and never take an issue with chronic fatigue, brain fog, or even depression.

We can also expect that all the other systems of our body are in well working order, and that nutrients of all sorts are being put to good use: not just for energy use, but for storage and "building up" tissues in the body that need more growth, development, or healing.

But, like any organ or gland in the body, the thyroid can dysfunction. For the thyroid specifically, this spells inevitable, slow dysfunction and even decline of many other physiological systems.

What are some of the ways this can happen? Let's take a look.

RT3 – Reverse Triidothyrinine

Going back to the thyroid hormones T3 and T4, **one of the biggest reasons for decreased thyroid**

ability is due to poor T4 to T3 conversion. There are many ways this can happen, which will be explored in the sections ahead. One thing to realize too about thyroid hormones, is that sometimes it's not just about poor conversion, but that **too much T4 is converted into "reverse T3" rather than regular T3.**

What's reverse T3 (RT3)? Unlike T4 or T3, RT3 is practically inactive as a hormone, and it is in fact released by the thyroid when it is sensed by the hypothalamus that thyroid activity should decrease. During all T4 conversion, it is said that 40% becomes T3, but the remaining 20% becomes RT3.

RT3 actually inhibits thyroid function, so if too much is converted to RT3, this can begin leading to an underactive thyroid. There are various things that can make RT3 conversion increase, which we'll look at throughout the chapter.

Pro-inflammatory Antibodies

Inflammation, in its very simplest definition, can be a source of damage and limitation of the thyroid. There are a wide range of triggers or causes to inflammation in the body itself that must be handled separately from the thyroid, in order to rein in harmful, chronic inflammation as the result of an immune system gone awry.

Some of the most common culprits for inflammation that can direct antibodies against the thyroid, however, are **overconsumption of inflammatory foods, or**

food intolerances and insensitivities (such as to gluten or dairy).

Bad sleeping habits are another element to consider, as poor sleep quality contributes to decreased immunity and heightened chronic inflammation. It is also very well known in the medical world that **auto-immune diseases**, huge creators of chronic inflammation, can lead attacks on the thyroid and cause some of the most common hypothyroid conditions that steal our energy and vitality.

Unhealthy Gut Microbiome

During T4 conversion into T3, some T4 doesn't "make it all the way"—instead being transformed into thyroid sulfates and acetic acids. These must then circulate down to the digestive system, where they are converted into more healthy, helpful T3, which "ups" thyroid function.

Clearly, if an unhealthy gut and weak digestive bacteria are prevalent, this can make way to diminished thyroid function and contribute to hypothyroid.

Poor Liver Function

Like the gut, the liver is instrumental to T4/T3 conversion. In fact, 80% of T4 produced gets sent down to the liver for processing, which is much more than what is sent to the digestive system. There in the liver, T4 is converted into either T3 or RT3.

If liver health is poor, then you can bet that thyroid health is poor. Toxins, hepatitis, chronic inflammation, alcohol use, and poor diet can slow down the liver's role in thyroid function, thus creating another undesirable gateway to hypothyroid problems.

Poor Nutrition

Certain dietary nutrients are essential for the thyroid to function correctly. The most commonly known one is **iodine, which the thyroid absolutely, 100% requires to synthesize both T3 and T4**.

In discussing thyroid treatment of any kind, wise and practiced health experts will always include iodine. **It is often little known (yet even statistically recorded by the World Health Organization) that iodine deficiency is one of the most common nutrient deficiencies plaguing the western population, no doubt participating in today's incredible prevalence of thyroid disease.**

Natural iodine was once present in soils all over the world. But due to widespread unsustainable agricultural practices, the trace element has been all but stripped from the earth, and now not abundantly present in the fruits and vegetables we eat. **For remedying an under-active thyroid disorder, some sufferers**

turn to trace amounts of iodine in seaweeds, kelps and iodized salts, though it is best to take iodine in the form of a supplement, which I will address in further detail later on in this book.

It is known too that low **iron** inhibits the thyroid, as it is useful in carrying the actual hormones to much-needed sites for energy usage. Low iron also causes anemia, which can compound the fatigue and listless symptoms of a hypothyroid.

It has also been surmised that lacking in **selenium, zinc, Omega-3's,** and **Vitamin D3** can play a role in underactive thyroid, although this is likely to be indirectly.

Stressful Lifestyle

Production of too much RT3 "de-activates" the thyroid, and one of the reasons for excessive RT3 can be connected to **too much biological stress**. Stress alone triggers a variety of bodily processes which, through one way or another, take hold on thyroid health.

High stress causes the release of **cortisol** from the adrenal glands, which in tandem lower the amount of available T3 by maintaining T4 levels. **Stress also encourages more synthesis of T4 into RT3, the inactive thyroid hormone.** There is so much T4 in the blood with excessive cortisol that the liver overcompensates, trying to desperately manage it by turning it into RT3.

Lower stress, and you increase thyroid function; too much stress, and this inhibits your thyroid, dwindling all the energy you need to life a happy, full life! Furthermore, it is incredibly important that you take adrenal health into consideration, and avoid adrenal depletion or fatigue.

Unstable Blood Sugar

Stable blood sugar is vital to correct immune response. If there is too much or too little, as in the case of Diabetes, this can have an effect on the thyroid and metabolism—while simultaneously ratcheting up poor, misfired immune reactions and chronic inflammation that, in turn, attacks the thyroid.

More and more evidence mounts with time that hypothyroid disorders and diabetes have some connection, with diabetes having to do with blood sugar dysfunction. Unstable blood sugar can lead to underactive thyroid, and then underactive thyroid contributes to yet more instability in blood sugar management sometimes—it's a vicious cycle.

The American Diabetes Association Journals cite a marked increase in the likelihood of hypothyroid dysfunction happening in those with Type 2 Diabetes, while also explaining that thyroid disorders make the management of blood glucose levels all the more difficult. A sluggish thyroid actually slows down the processing of blood sugars and even diabetic medications, which can create dangerous drops in blood sugar!

Genetic Factors

Studies by the European Department of Endocrinology confirm that **one of the most likely precursors to thyroid dysfunction is genetics**. The likelihood of developing a hypothyroid disorder could largely depend on the genes you inherit from your ancestors, especially if genetics in your family show a tendency of having auto-immune diseases. These direct chronic inflammation at healthy tissues, one target possibly being the thyroid gland itself.

At an even deeper level, unhealthy mitochondrial function in the cells can lead to hypothyroid, which is also rooted in genetics. If mitochondria (an integral part of cell function) are not operating due to their genetic coding, underactive thyroid problems might slowly develop, as a consequence.

Mitochondria dysfunction can also contribute to heightened levels of inflammation that attack the thyroid, as it is connected to genetics and auto-immune diseases as well.

Conventional Hyperthyroid Treatments

On the opposite end of the spectrum from Hypothyroid

are Hyperthyroid problems, for which modern medicine has a variety of approaches to treatment. Hyperthyroidism happens when the thyroid is much TOO active, which comes with its own long list of problems.

Unfortunately, some of Hyperthyroid treatments involve radiation or medication that drives thyroid function down, sometimes permanently. There are also surgeries to remove the thyroid completely, just to bring a Hyperthyroid back to healthier function.

What happens in some cases instead is the creation of Hypothyroidism, which must then be managed in its own way. **In summary, some conventional approaches to thyroid disorders are actually the cause of yet more disorders!**

This is why it is absolutely important for patients and sufferers of thyroid issues to educate and empower themselves, as some conventional approaches can sometimes lack sound solutions or adequate understanding of a person's specific thyroid hormone levels and history. Naturally supporting and healing your own thyroid can be the very best frontline defense!

In the chapters so far, we have discussed all angles of viewing the thyroid and how it works: including when the thyroid is at its prime, but also what can cause it to lose strength and function, thus creating poor health, diminished energy, and worsened quality of life.

Becoming acquainted with the thyroid's interconnectedness to other conditions, illnesses,

and other bodily systems as well, can help us further grasp what elements of our health to keep an eye on, and create hopeful solutions. There are many symptoms of a slowly diminishing thyroid to watch out for, as well as a long list of illnesses that could themselves be thyroid disorders—either that, or diseases that an underactive thyroid might contribute to.

What are they, you might ask? For the next chapter, all of that will be sorted through and examined in as simple a way possible. **Read on, as we begin to delve into the more specific medical terminology and pathology of hypothyroid health: including diseases and symptoms related to the illness.**

CHAPTER 4

Symptoms and Conditions of Hypothyroidism

Now that we know the basics of thyroid function—at its best, and at its worst—the next best step in understanding its issues is in getting acquainted with signs and symptoms of developing thyroid disorders. As hypothyroid can sometimes be a subtle change in health at best, it can also be a difficult condition to pinpoint and diagnose.

The more knowledge of its conditions and symptoms, the better equipped you will be in determining whether or not you have a thyroid problem. **It's important to note, however, that some of the following symptoms and conditions do *NOT* mean that you have a thyroid problem for sure.** Even someone with all of the tell-tale signs of an underactive thyroid may in fact have a completely different network of issues going on, which is why it is important that you turn to other resources in determining the real underlying issue.

Still, that doesn't mean it's a bad idea that they get their thyroid checked out by a health practitioner to eliminate the possibility.

Together with the following sections on Hypothyroid Symptoms and Related Conditions, I would recommend that anyone strongly consider various lab tests available for checking on their thyroid, if they are suspecting any problems.

There are a few things to take into account regarding many modern lab tests for detecting thyroid problems, however. Some tests are made only to detect levels of T4, or TSH (thyroid stimulating hormone). When these are found in high or low amounts, a doctor might feel impelled to diagnose you with a thyroid disorder, or they could overlook the possibility of you having one, based on the numbers they see in the tests.

However, levels of T4 or TSH don't say enough about your thyroid levels. **When looking into testing, do make sure that you find doctors or practitioners who also test for T3 and RT3 levels.** It is arguable that these are the numbers to really look out for: as you could have tons of circulating T4 (which seems healthy), but not as much converted T3, which is much more important.

Further, **a test comparing a T3 to RT3 ratio** might help determine whether or not you have enough of the "more powerful" hormone to keep your thyroid function healthy. There are also tests that scan for anti-thyroid **antibodies**, which could signal that you have an inflammatory immune disorder and an immune system that is attacking your thyroid—a classic sign of some specific thyroid conditions.

Iodine Testing – Just as Important!

After thyroid hormone tests, **iodine tests** are choice at determining the severity of hypothyroid symptoms. Considering that **iodine deficiency** is one of the leading nutritional causes for hypothyroidism, and that iodine can in fact be tested for, having levels of this important element checked could be an important step in finding answers to your thyroid troubles!

In fact, iodine is very important to check for, as *some forms of hypothyroidism cannot be detected by thyroid hormone tests alone.* **Further, a doctor might not even diagnose you as hypothyroid if the thyroid hormone levels they test appear in a stable range, sometimes failing to truly reflect the thyroid disorder at hand.**

As such, consider asking for an iodine test. Some (but unfortunately not all) healthcare practitioners are proficient and literate in these tests, specifically if you ask for a **24 hour iodine loading test** (urine), which is the best way to determine your iodine levels and can also be ordered easily and comfortably in your own home through various clinical services online.

Otherwise, some doctors might tell you "you don't have hypothyroidism!" if you don't have your iodine levels checked. Make sure to take that into consideration—especially if you are suffering from obvious, defined hypothyroid systems, and doctor after doctor can only tell you: "Nope—tests are showing nothing. It must all be in your head."

Diagnosis or no, the following sections on Symptoms and Conditions can help you further determine if you need tests. **The next chapter altogether, on Remedies and Strategies, can help also help you support and heal your thyroid naturally—whether you have been officially diagnosed as hypothyroid, or not!**

The Basal Body Temperature Test – Simple, But Eye-Opening

Use this simple at-home test to get a gauge on your thyroid health—and help you make the decision to get further testing, and find more answers about whether you truly have hypothyroidism.

Using either a Mercury (preferred) or Digital Thermometer, **one checks their body temperature at choice points throughout the day** (oral or armpit). **The most suspect points of the day are immediately in the morning after you wake up and are still in bed, and "mid-afternoon," around 3 PM.** Temperature must be taken several times for several days, over an extended period of time, to get an accurate judge of "consistency" and a long-term, below-normal basal body temperature that hints at hypothyroidism.

If during the morning test your body temperature is between 97.8 and 98.2 degrees Fahrenheit, your thyroid health is most likely normal. But if it is lower, this could indicate slowed metabolism, and hypothyroid. **If the mid-afternoon body temperature, too, is low—98.5 degrees Fahrenheit or lower—this is also a sign of possible hypothyroidism**, especially if you receive these low temperatures consistently over many, many days.

Try the basal body temperature test to see what it tells you. If it's pointing to low temperature, and thus low metabolism—consider further testing, to see a doctor, or for further clues about hypothyroidism.

The following symptoms and conditions can help you pinpoint possible underactive thyroid levels, too.

Symptoms of a Hypothyroid Condition

- **Fatigue** – at the cellular level, energy usage slows down with an underactive thyroid. This leads to fatigue, lethargy, and unrestful sleep, no matter how much.

- **"Brain Fog," Inability to Think Clearly, Memory Problems** – an active thyroid is key to optimal brain function, as it allocates proteins to brain tissue.

- **Depression or Changeable Mood** – as thyroid is connected to brain function, the actions of neurotransmitters fail—leading to depression and "low moods."

• **Cold Sensitivity** – cardiac output lowers with less thyroid hormones, decreasing circulation and basal body temperature, thus giving the "chills."

• **Dry Skin** – the thyroid regulates sweat and sebaceous glands in the skin. When underactive, the skin dries up, and there might be related sweating problems.

• **Weight Gain, Bloated or "Puffy" Appearance** – since metabolism slows down, more weight is put on, even if appetite is relatively low.

• **Hair Loss** – thyroid hormones stimulate hair growth. When lacking, hair loss may ensue, due to lack of action from thyroid-dependent sebaceous glands.

• **Slower Heart Rate** – thyroid hormones increase heart rate. When absent, heart rate slows down, especially if there are high levels of RT3.

• **Constipation** – effects of hypothyroid can be felt in the gut. Gut dysfunction can also be a cause of hypothyroid, but overall, all digestive actions slow down.

• **Irregular, Heavy Periods with Strong Mood Changes** – thyroid hormones stimulate too much progestin vs. estrogen, leading to heavy periods/ irritability.

• **Joint or Muscle Pain** – with a low thyroid, crucial minerals like calcium and magnesium are poorly processed, leading to body pains, aches, and cramps.

• **High Cholesterol** – as metabolism slows with low thyroid, harmful LDL cholesterol circulates more in the blood, as it fails to be metabolized quickly.

• **Enlarged Thyroid Gland, or "Goiter"** – this can sometimes even be felt or seen. Goiter can be associated with a hyperthyroid, and in extreme cases, the thyroid can be seen as a swollen growth in the neck. However, in both hypothyroid and auto-immune thyroid issues, *a goiter can indicate a severe iodine deficiency, and that the thyroid is enlarging to trap as much iodine as possible—or that the thyroid is "inflamed" from too many auto-immune antibodies attacking its tissues.*

Hypothyroid Conditions

• **Thyroiditis** – there are many different kinds of thyroiditis, which are characterized by inflammation of the thyroid for one reason or another.

• **Hashimoto's Thyroiditis** – the most common type of thyroiditis. It is the archetype hypothyroid auto-immune disease, with antibodies attacking healthy tissues not just in the thyroid, but in the entire body.

• **Thyroid Nodules** – typically harmless growths on the thyroid gland. However, they can inhibit or interfere with thyroid function.

• **Thyroid Cancer** – a less common cancer of the thyroid, often quite small and mostly treatable. Symptoms of thyroid cancer can include diminished function.

• **Myxedema Coma** – complete loss of brain

function, but only after years of constant, severely low levels of thyroid hormone. It is relatively rare, and can be prevented easily if levels of thyroid hormones are managed.

Conditions Related to Hypothyroidism

• **Hypertension** – cardiac output decreases with lowered thyroid, making the heart have to work harder to move blood: thus raising blood pressure.

• **Obesity** – metabolism can slow almost to a halt with hypothyroidism, and it can take little for a sufferer to gain excessive weight or even become obese.

• **Vitiligo** – an auto-immune skin disease, involving the dysfunction of cells responsible for producing "melanin"/skin color, may coincide with hypothyroid.

• **Hypercholesterolemia (High Cholesterol)** – metabolizing of cholesterol slows. Those with hypothyroid could have dangerously high cholesterol levels.

• **Celiac Disease** – unmanaged Celiac, an auto-immune intolerance of gluten, can create harmful inflammatory antibodies that attack and deplete the thyroid.

• **Auto-Immune Diseases** – various auto-immune illnesses of all types can be connected to hypothyroid: including rheumatoid arthritis or lupus, for example.

- **Clinical Depression** – hypothyroidism can influence neurotransmitter disorders, sometimes pushing sufferers into the zone of more severe depressions.

- **Fibromyalgia** – if hypothyroidism is connected to poor sleeping habits and lack of processed calcium and magnesium, fibromyalgia could very well be connected.

- **Chronic Fatigue Syndrome** – this mysterious syndrome has many suspected causes, not the least of which being hypothyroidism, among other disorders.

- **Heart Disease** – hypothyroid can encourage high blood pressure and high cholesterol, which thus increases the risk of heart disease or attack.

The underactive function of a thyroid gland leads the way to many various symptoms and possible illnesses. Some of them are directly related to the thyroid—others arise in different body systems as the result of failing thyroid hormone function.

Next, we'll be moving on to ways that hypothyroid can be treated. There are a variety of methods that doctors use to treat hypothyroidism once low thyroid hormones are detected, such as iodine radiation, thyroid hormone replacement, medication, and even thyroid surgery: very dramatic, expensive, and sometimes even dangerous operations for health.

Fortunately for you, this book is full of the good stuff: only natural, gentle ways of handling a

suspected underactive thyroid.

If you think you might have a diagnosable hypothyroidism problem, I can only recommend testing by
a doctor, and that you seek his or her treatment and
advice. **I must emphasize also that none of the
information in this book is intended to diagnose or recommend cure against a hypothyroid
disorder.**

However, with the approval of your physician, the next
chapter is full of many remedies and approaches I have
studied. Each can help heal and support thyroid function naturally. It's up to you to research, decide, or
discuss with your physician which approaches are right
for you. These can consist of foods, diet tips, lifestyle
advice, and even herbal remedies to help you regain that
energy and find the healing you've been looking for.

Even if you don't have a hypothyroid disorder, soak in
or even try some of the following chapter's strategies
and information: whether you are just concerned about
preventing and holding off an underactive thyroid, or
you want to learn new and natural ways to support your
own hypothyroid disorder—or a disorder in someone
you love.

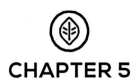

CHAPTER 5

20+ Remedies for Healing Hypothyroidism Naturally

We're now at the best part of the book, and understanding hypothyroidism in general! The following chapter is chock-full of **over 20 remedies, tips, foods, herbs, and strategies** to maintaining and keeping your thyroid healthy, which could be incredibly useful if permitted and approved by your own doctor.

Please peruse the next few pages and use what you will. Each contains information based off my own research, experience, and recommendation from health professionals, too. **I've used this information to help myself and others manage, prevent, and even battle against hypothyroid issues, to recover stolen energy and life quality. Now you can, too!**

Do remember that none of these strategies or remedies are a 'quick-fix' cure for hypothyroid, and if you do suspect you have an underactive thyroid issue, don't be afraid to talk to your physician as well as discuss natural methods to support conventional treatments.

Increase Iodine in Your Diet

Making sure you get enough dietary iodine, a trace

element found in some foods, cannot be stressed enough. Iodine is absolutely necessary for the production of thyroid hormones T3 and T4. Without it, the thyroid ails, and can especially lean towards the hypo-thyroid end of the spectrum.

Iodine deficiency is inaccurately perceived to be an uncommon problem, as in most regions some foods contain small amounts of added iodine through table or sea salt—this being just enough to avoid the enlargement of the thyroid (goiter), but simply not enough for optimal thyroid function.

Iodine deficiency problems are rampant around the globe today, and are highly misunderstood in mainstream medicine. With time, it is becoming clear that iodized salts are not enough of a solution to iodine depletion.

Today, parts of the U.S. and Australia are somewhat vulnerable to iodine deficiency. But some health studies (along with the World Health Organization statistics) document that **populations in Europe, Latin America, Asia, and Africa are rapidly becoming more and more iodine depleted, and of growing serious concern: especially in developing countries.**

Obviously, iodine is quite important—and iodized salts are not enough for some populations. **Besides table or sea salt, however, what foods can you look for to find your iodine sources?**

Seaweed and kelps are popularly considered good

iodine-rich foods. But with concerns for a recent increase in arsenic levels in these plant foods, depending on them solely for iodine intake has raised some questions about implementing them into your daily diet for iodine supplementation—and the harms they could create.

Other common plant sources of trace iodine are **corn, prunes, lima beans, apples, green peas, potatoes, strawberries and cranberries**. **Watercress** is an aquatic vegetable, both wild and cultivated, that boasts great levels of iodine. Consider seeking it out or foraging it as a wild edible to get adequate amounts of this element into your diet.

You may use a little table or iodized salt each day, which can add to your required iodine intake, but can fail to make up for all that you need for some suffering from hypothyroidism.

For those with more severe iodine deficiencies, however, **iodine supplements** are the only effective approach in some cases. These supplements should contain both **iodine and iodide**, which together are required to fully support the body's ability to synthesize its own thyroid hormones, and are *absolutely* necessary for healing a thyroid that is certainly underactive. Salts, foods, and other iodine sources are of little help compared to supplements.

The American Thyroid Association recommends a daily allowance of 150 mcg a day for adults, which may be fine if you have already sufficient iodine levels. But for those with an underactive thyroid, the allowance might be much more,

depending on your levels and physician's recommendations. I recommend seeking an iodine-literate practitioner whom can help devise a personalized protocol that is right for you, alongside supplementing with other companion nutrients for the best synergistic results.

Here is an essential web link for further reading about the importance of iodine, with a list of helpful references:

www.stopthethyroidmadness.com/iodine12345

Foods with Selenium

Modern research is beginning to target selenium as one of the second most important trace minerals for functioning thyroid, after iodine. In trials undergone by the Journal of Clinical Endocrinology on those with auto-immune hypothyroid issues (like Hashimoto's), there was demonstrated improvement of auto-immune issues if selenium uptake was increased—and especially if they had a selenium deficiency in the first place!

Selenium is a trace, dietary element that can be found in high amounts from plant sources actively incorporated into your diet! If you eat the following foods regularly, along with a diet relatively high in plants and vegetables, your selenium needs will be taken care of.

The recommended daily allowance for selenium is 55 to 75 mcg per day (not to exceed 200mcg)

and can be obtained through brazil nuts, many other types of nuts (pecans, walnuts, almonds—not peanuts), mushrooms, asparagus and sunflower seeds. One brazil nut contains about 200 mcg, so eat them once in a while.

Boost Up Your Vitamins (A, B, C, D, and E)

Apparently, most vitamins are strongly linked and even necessary to certain thyroid processes. A handful of vitamins are **antioxidants**, which help stave off free radicals in the body—harmful cell development that can eventually hurt the thyroid.

In fact, a lot of free radicals are created through the interactions between thyroid hormones and cells themselves, making plenty of vitamin nutrition important!

Vitamin A – An antioxidant, prevents oxidative stress during metabolism via thyroid hormones. Vitamin A also boosts iodine uptake by the thyroid, and encourages healthy secretion of TSH to trigger T3 and T4 release.

Vitamin A-rich plant sources include: Carrots, acorn squash, pumpkin, sweet potatoes, cantaloupe, sweet peppers, apricots, naturally "orange" foods, dark leafy greens. Recommended daily allowance is between 700 and 900 mcg per day.

Vitamin B – Vitamins B6 and B12 are also highly important thyroid vitamins. These are "co-enzymes," rather than antioxidants, instrumental to protein and hormone process all over the body.

B6 (or pyridoxine) has been observed as a part of the release of thyrotropin-releasing hormone (TRH), the hormone that first triggers the pituitary gland before it then triggers the thyroid—making it of prime importance!

Plant foods rich in B6: Potatoes, sweet potatoes, carrots, prunes, vegemite, avocadoes, bananas, plantains, soy, pinto beans, lentil beans, pistachios. The recommended daily allowance for B6 is between 1 and 2 mg, and not to exceed 100 mg per day (in supplement form).

B12 (cobalamin) might be deficient in thyroid disorders, which often manifests as gastritis or a digestive disorder. Research and studies are not clear, however, whether B12 contributes to thyroid issues, or whether thyroid issues contribute to B12 deficiency. Either way, count vitamin B12 as important!

Plants high in B12: Turn to nutritional yeast, vegemite, soy, shiitake/chanterelle/lion's mane mushrooms, tea (green, black, oolong), or B12 fortified and healthy foods. Alternatively you may wish to take a supplement to cover your B12 needs. The recommended daily allowance for B12 is between 2 and 3 mcg, or more if you discover you are deficient.

Vitamin C – A bit like vitamin A, C is an antioxidant and very important during the metabolizing process. It rids the body of free radicals, which can quickly oxidize and interfere with future efforts of cell energy use.

Foods high in vitamin C: Citrus (oranges, lemon, lime, grapefruit), strawberries, cranberries, blueberries, raspberries, rosehips. The recommended daily allowance for Vitamin C is between 46 and 60 mg per day, to prevent "scurvy" or vitamin-C deficiency.

Vitamin D – D3 is specifically key to thyroid health, especially if auto-immune issues and inflammation are suspected. Low amounts of D3 have been detected in those with thyroid disorders. It wouldn't be a bad idea to focus on supplementation, if you suspect that you're not getting enough—and a good amount of the population doesn't!

Plant foods high in vitamin D: Mushrooms, such as shiitake or portobello. Plant derived vitamin D supplements are also helpful; however, exposing the skin to sunlight for 20-30 minutes/day provides the highest sources of accessible vitamin D. The recommended daily allowance is 600 IU (international units) for below-70-aged adults.

Vitamin E – An antioxidant like vitamins A or C, vitamin E helps prevent oxidative stress during the course of energy metabolism. Trials with vitamin E showed that supplementation improved dysfunction in both hypo- and hyper-thyroid disorders.

Plant foods rich in E are abundant: Most nuts and seeds, such as sunflower, peanuts and almonds (including butters made from these), spinach, beets, chard, safflower, pumpkin, red peppers, mangoes, avocadoes. The recommended daily allowance of vitamin E is 15 mg/day.

Studies by the Journal of Nutrition found that depletion of magnesium in the diet could lend itself to decreased production of T4 thyroid hormone. Furthermore, zinc has also been linked with boosting healthy levels of **free-circulating T3**, a form of powerful thyroid hormone that remains unbound to proteins in the blood—thus making it much easier for uptake, and keeping metabolism levels healthy and optimal.

Zinc and magnesium together have also been linked to mediating healthy levels of inflammation in the body, so getting adequate amounts of these minerals could help stave off the harms of auto-antibodies to the thyroid, such as in Hashimoto's Thyroiditis: an auto-immune condition.

Plant sources rich in magnesium: Swiss chard, purslane, spinach, beets, nopal cactus, amaranth, quinoa, arugula, okra. The recommended daily allowance of magnesium is currently in between 100 and 400 mg per day.

Plant sources rich in zinc: Endive, pumpkins, gourds, mushrooms (crimini, e.g), alfalfa sprouts, zucchini, bamboo shoots, broccoli, epazote. Recommended daily zinc allowance is from 8 mg to 11 mg per day.

Try Some L-Tyrosine in Natural Foods

Like iodine, **L-tyrosine** (an amino acid) is crucial to the synthesis of thyroid hormones T3 and T4. It is found in a number of common foods that, if not implemented into a versatile healthy diet, could have an impact on thyroid health and function in some ways.

However, it is important for those experiencing hypothyroid issues to **avoid supplementation of L-tyrosine**, even if a doctor, practitioner, nutritionist, or health store manager recommends it as a way to treat hypothyroidism. ***The Journal of Clinical Investigation* published findings showing that l-tyrosine, in synthetic clinical doses, actually *suppresses* thyroid activity: binding to iodine and in fact making the body lose more of it than with low iodine levels alone.**

As such, simply consider whether or not you are including foods containing L-Tyrosine regularly in your diet. **Plant sources range from soy, peanuts, and almonds to avocadoes, bananas, lima beans, pumpkin seeds, and sesame seeds.** If these foods are lacking, try to incorporate a few more of them—but do not view them as a way to treat hypothyroid.

Of note: for the most part, L-Tyrosine is already taken in and produced in adequate levels naturally by the body for healthy function.

Avoid "Super-Antioxidants" Like Co-enzyme Q10 or Glutathione

Like antioxidant vitamins, certain other antioxidants and free-radical fighters are significant to the function of the thyroid in the body. Examples like **Co-enzyme Q10** and **Glutathione** are talked about often in relation to hypothyroidism, with some people condoning or purchasing products and supplements rich in these helpful oxidative stress-busters—all with hopes to beat the disorder naturally.

For those curious about the antioxidant science behind thyroid health: **Co-enzyme Q10 and Glutathione are produced, raised, and lowered naturally by the body.** Their levels actually reflect the strength of the body's anti-oxidative system, with these two anti-oxidants fluctuating naturally depending on the body's needs.

Like L-Tyrosine, certain health practitioners might condone supplementation of these two antioxidants, but this can be ineffective on hypothyroid health. In fact, *The International Journal of Molecular Sciences* **observed that increased levels of Co-enzyme Q10 happens naturally in the body when it experiences lack of thyroid hormones or iodine.**

Supplementation, as a result, is being questioned by many health authorities. Some even wonder if taking Co-enzyme Q10 could be of harm to hypothyroidism, if the body produces so many of these circulating antioxidants already.

Glutathione, on the other hand, is also given in supplement form—**but dietary supplement experts find that glutathione in supplement form does nothing to boost the levels that the body already makes**, as the gut is simply not strong enough to process and absorb glutathione in a pill.

Dr. Shawn Talbott, PhD and published dietary supplement expert, says that **the only way to support healthy Co-enzyme Q10 and Glutathione levels is to support the anti-oxidative-immune system itself.** How can you achieve this? By eating other easily-digestible antioxidant boosters like Vitamin A, C, or E.

Eat More Omega-3's

Omega-3 fatty acids are long-chain, polyunsaturated fats that help mediate inflammation throughout the body, and specifically have some impact on brain function by ameliorating chronic, harmful inflammation. Thyroid health, too, has established a strong link to brain health and mental function as well.

Together, optimum thyroid hormones and healthy fats are great catalysts against poor energy use, fatigue, inflammation, and poor mental function associated with hypothyroid—**and in fact, supplementation of Omega-3 has been shown to be therapeutic and helpful in reducing cognitive symptoms and**

complications of hypothyroidism, in an Egyptian study published in their Physiology Journal.

Omega-3's reduce oxidative stress naturally as well, much like vitamin antioxidants, and thus are altogether highly impactful against immune/inflammation-oriented complications connected to hypothyroid—including Hashimoto's. Consider Omega-3's specifically if you have auto-immune issues related to hypothyroid, or if you struggle with brain fog, fatigue, and poor concentration.

Natural Plant Sources of Omega-3 Fatty Acids: Flax seed, chia seeds, almonds, avocados, purslane, evening primrose oil, pumpkin seeds.

The World Health Organization recommends a daily EPA (Eicosapentaenoic Acid) and DHA (Docosahexaenoic Acid) intake of 0.3-0.5 grams, and a daily ALA (Alpha-linolenic Acid) intake of 0.8-1.1 grams—each of these acids being different "chains" of Omega-3.

Skip the Inflammatory Foods

"Inflammatory Foods" are pervasive and numerous, a category that includes most foods commonly perceived to be unhealthy in general. These promote chronic inflammation all throughout the body, the consequence of a confused or misfiring immune system.

As we have discussed previously in this book, auto-immune issues can be the direct cause, or a main participant in, certain hypothyroid disorders. **Hashimoto's is the most common auto-immune hypothyroid issue, while also being one of the leading disorders of hypothyroidism, period.**

Auto-immune disorders create anti-bodies that attack the body's healthy cells and tissues, while promoting harmful levels of chronic inflammation. As such, implementing a diet low (or complete void) in inflammatory foods can have a hand in helping reduce the unhealthy, auto-immune inflammation that can destroy the thyroid in illnesses like Hashimoto's.

Basic inflammatory foods to avoid: Animal proteins (meat, eggs, dairy), processed foods, fried/deep fried foods, foods with additives/enrichments (high fructose corn syrup, MSG, food dyes, added vitamins), harmful fats (trans/saturated), refined sugars, and gluten products (wheat, rye, barley).

If you want to learn more about harmful inflammation itself and how to manage it, I would highly suggest you explore this in my other book, *Natural Anti-Inflammatory Remedies.*

Herbal Remedies for Thyroid Function

Certain herbs, supplements, and remedies can AND **do** work for supporting an underactive thyroid. Talk with your doctor, and consult with an herbalist/expert in botanical medicine before considering inclusion of these in addition to your diet or medications.

• **Ashwagandha (Withania somnifera)** – contains high levels of magnesium and iron, which helps proliferation of T4 and the transfer of thyroid hormones to needed sites through the bloodstream. Can be a useful, nutritional and therapeutic booster in those with hypothyroidism and deficient in these two important minerals. Ashwagandha has been known to boost thyroid hormone levels.

Avoid use of Ashwagandha if pregnant, nursing, or if you have low blood pressure, nightshade allergies, or are using certain diabetic medications.

• **Burdock (Arctium lappa)** – This culinary root in Oriental cuisine has been used as a "liver detoxifier," helping the digestive system speed up the eliminations of toxins and waste. It also enhances gut motility and digestive function in general. Consider incorporating it as a food or in medicinal amounts for liver support, if you suspect a sluggish liver might be a part of your underactive thyroid symptoms.

Avoid excessive use, especially if pregnant.

• **Milk Thistle (Silybum marianum)** – This remarkable plant contains silymarins, compounds that block toxin entrance into the liver while also acting as antioxidants. These compounds are entirely unique to the Milk Thistle plant. It has also been seen to speed the natural recovery, healing, and growth of new, healthy liver cells—hence supporting liver health, which is vital to thyroid hormone conversion, an important asset to a healthy thyroid.

Milk Thistle could support a damaged liver contributing to hypothyroid disease. *Use only in directed amounts, and discontinue use if you have stomach upset, diarrhea, or an allergic reaction.*

• **Rosemary (Rosmarinus officinalis)** – Rosemary's active constituent, rosemarinic acid, is a powerful antioxidant that could help reduce oxidative stress linked to thyroid functions. Think of it as a powerful fighter, alongside common food-antioxidants like vitamins A, C, and E.

To top it all off, Rosemary opens circulation and improves blood flow, known to help with brain and mental function struggles associated with symptoms of hypothyroidism.

Do not ingest Rosemary essential oils, and discontinue any preparations of Rosemary if they cause stomach upset or kidney irritation. Do not use excessive amounts of the plant, as it can be toxic.

• **Green Tea (Camellia sinensis)** – This lovely hot beverage plant can be found in practically every grocery store, and touts amazingly high levels of antioxidants that could help support underactive thyroid functions. Consider a brew a day if you have hypothyroidism and you suspect you don't get enough anti-oxidants in your diet.

Green Tea also contains caffeine. Large amounts can cause jitteriness, anxiety, stomach upset and heart rate increase. Pregnant women should avoid consuming it in high amounts.

• **Licorice (Glycyrrhiza glabra)** – A powerful immune agent, Licorice is chock-full of iron, magnesium, and antioxidants all together. It has been helpful as a treatment for underactive thyroid that might be the result of a depleted immune system, or poor diet.

It is a sweet, smooth root with a pleasant taste, and can often be purchased at tea shops or health food stores. Cautiously, it could be used to treat auto-immune Hashimoto's, but only a practitioner will be able to determine if Licorice will be helpful or not.

Generally, avoid use if you have auto-immune issues, as Licorice is known to activate even an overactive immune system—making anti-thyroid antibodies even more damaging.

Also avoid use if you are pregnant, have high blood pressure, and a risk of diabetes, heart attack or stroke. Avoid eating in daily excessive amounts.

Digestive Health: A Must

Back in Chapter 1, the conversion from T4 into T3 was described: a process turning a mostly inactive, but highly plentiful thyroid hormone (T4) into a much more useful one (T3). **The gut is responsible for converting about 20% of T4 into much needed T3 for optimal metabolism and energy.**

If your digestive health is awful, then you can bet that your thyroid levels are being affected. Your intestines, filled with millions of active, pro-biotic bacteria, are what help your body produce the T3 levels you need to have a stable thyroid, as opposed to an underactive one. Ensuring that your digestive system is up-to-par for thyroid health depends on many factors. **We've touched on a few of these factors already: avoid inflammatory foods, and eat an impeccable diet,** as that will also influence the health of your digestive tract.

Fiber from plant foods is especially important, along with getting an adequate introduction of fresh, strong new probiotics from fermented foods like sauerkraut, kombucha, or kimchi.

Want the whole scoop on gut health? I'd suggest another one of my popular reads: *Healthy Gut Solution*, which discusses and explores all the different levels of naturally healing your digestive system, along with many useful methods and tips!

Liver Health and Detox

After your gut (and specifically your intestines), your liver is the second-most important organ for helping with thyroid processes. 20% of T4 is converted into T3 by a healthy gut microbiome. **Another 60% depends on the liver for conversion into the T3 levels our bodies need.**

Overburdening the liver can thus be a source of frustrating and debilitating thyroid symptoms, so focusing on its health can lead to positive change. Consider supporting toxin elimination with the use of certain herbs *(see Herbal Remedies section)*, or **incorporating vegetables with affinities to the liver: such as beets, daikon radishes, dandelion, celery and artichoke.** Avoiding inflammatory foods and too many animal proteins can also help.

If you are drinking too much alcohol or over-exposing yourself to certain harmful, environmental toxins or chemicals **(such as herbicides, pesticides, pollution, cleaners, xenoestrogens, smoke)**, then try to reduce those factors—they could be preventing your liver from doing its job!

Support Your Immune System

This goes back to auto-immune issues and inflammation once again, an issue that cannot be overlooked enough. Various studies from multiple disciplines have shown, time and time again, that immune dysfunction can have a hand in hypothyroidism—and specifically the most common cause for the disorder, the auto-immune **Hashimoto's Thyroiditis**.

An immune system that is out-of-whack can be one of the many toppling factors in a physiological domino-effect leading to hypothyroidism. *Support your immune function by considering many or all of the previously addressed strategies:* **avoid inflammatory foods,**

increase your anti-oxidant intake, get some healthy exercise, and make sure you are getting all the nutrition that you need!

All of these can help prevent your body from creating chronic inflammation and disparaging antibodies, influences that slowly destroy and inflame the thyroid. **But are there other approaches to immune system support?** The following strategies are also immune-boosting, while promoting excellent thyroid and overall health.

Food Intolerances? Eliminate Them!

Food intolerances and hypersensitivities wreak havoc on both the immune system and digestive system alike. Not only can exposure to food sensitivities wreck the digestive microbiome, but it can rev-up our immune systems to be "overactive," training them to attack and react in ways that damage perfectly normal tissues, and spread chronic inflammation.

A faulty immune system attacks the thyroid; a dysfunctional gut reduces the conversion of T4 into T3. Is ignoring the fact that you might have a food intolerance a good idea, if you think you have hypothyroid symptoms? The answer is: **absolutely not!**

Consider that you could have a food intolerance if some of the tell-tale symptoms of hypothyroidism are cropping up, especially if there are digestive issues and if you are diagnosed with Hashimoto's. Even get testing if you have suspicions about certain foods. **Sensitivities (and even food allergies) to wheat, gluten, beans, nightshades, dairy, and other foods could be cranking up your immune system, and causing it to attack your thyroid.**

This extends to **Celiac disease**, a digestive/immune disorder that if undiagnosed, can create all sorts of autoimmune issues all over the body: not just Hashimoto's Thyroiditis, but possibly Rheumatoid Arthritis, Lupus, Vitiligo, and other auto-immune disorders as well.

Reduce Stress

There is too much evidence to ignore stress in the case of supporting one's immune system. Yes, stress—through immune function—can have an impact on thyroid levels, causing them to plummet if stressful chemicals are rampant much too often throughout the body and the brain.

Stress reduces immune function, it's true—experts at the Mayo Clinic state "[stress] alters immune system responses, and suppresses the digestive system, reproductive system, and growth processes." In multiple ways, these all affect thyroid hormone levels, causing the immune system to attack the thyroid in some cases.

Stress increases the release of cortisol and adrenaline from the adrenal glands. **Cortisol has been known to inhibit the conversion of T4 into needed T3, while stifling hormone-receptor sensitivity to**

free-floating T3. Cortisol also raises levels of RT3, a thyroid hormone that is inactive and in fact, suppresses thyroid function, if anything.

That's why stress, and even adrenal health, are not to be forgotten—both for direct thyroid care and immune system support in general. If you'd like the skinny on adrenal health and healing your adrenal gland from the fatigue and depletion of too much stress, try another one of my books, *Adrenal Fatigue: Cure It Naturally*.

Sleep Well

Sleep is deeply rooted in stress, immune health, and hence, thyroid function. An often overlooked (even skipped!) part of our daily lives, we must all take the time to examine whether or not we are getting the adequate sleep to regulate some of our body's most important processes.

Recent observational studies bare evidence that 8 hours of sleep or more is the most optimal on average for human adults. 7 hours or less, and people begin to experience lowered immunity: higher incidences of colds, allergies, and a general feeling of malaise and fatigue. Further, people who don't get enough sleep are 3 times more likely to catch common illnesses, like the common cold, thus revealing diminished immune strength and robustness.

The connection can easily be made that those who form terrible sleeping habits could be at risk of heightened, harmful immune responses, which could in turn damage the thyroid. While lack of, or poor, sleep is definitely not a single cause for auto-immune disorders like Hashimoto's Thyroiditis, no doubt continuing with less-than-healthy sleep habits makes symptoms and suffering worse.

Sleep, stress, and diet are all great contributors to immune health. Immune health contributes to thyroid health. While boosting your immune system, by various means, is not a direct cure from plummeted levels of thyroid hormone—abandoning your immune health is no help on that count, and could in fact be an important stepping stone in getting your thyroid health and energy levels back on track!

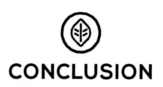

CONCLUSION

Thank you, again, for purchasing and reading *Thyroid Support*. If you appreciate the information or have learned anything fresh and useful in the process, then I feel honored by you—and I consider one of my many goals as a writer, health-lover and educator complete!

I hope that my experiences and research have given you some invaluable ideas and tips you can use to forgo a whole new path, through the complex world that is thyroid health. There is a lot of information out there: I have done my very best, with all honesty in my search for the truth and essence at the core of hypothyroidism, to help give you a primer you can then use to find yet more truth and information on the subject.

Who knows, maybe it will even carry you through to the resolution and healing of your own thyroid issues, or the issues your loved ones are experiencing.

Hypothyroidism symptoms can be confusing and over-whelming. If you do feel lost in a sea of differing opinions, facts, and approaches—or even those symptoms of fatigue, lethargy, brain fog, weight gain, or worse—you can always turn to this book for comfort and knowledge again, a place to "start-over" or reset in your search for health and truth again.

Remember: always use herbs and supplements in a cautious, informed way. **Knowledge is power, and if you are ever in doubt about the state of your health and if hypothyroidism is playing a role— never hesitate to contact a professional health practitioner who can help you with these issues, and narrow down a cause or diagnosis.** This is especially important if you fear that you could have a major hypothyroid disorder, like Thyroid Cancer or Hashimoto's.

I will leave you here, but stay connected and in touch with my *Carma Books* community for more books on holistic, natural, and plant-based health. Reach out again soon for more forthcoming, much-talked-about health titles, along with plenty of experiences and sharing of tips and knowledge on how to empower healing in your own life—and to get the most mileage out of your health potential!

A WORD FROM THE PUBLISHER

Hi, I'm Carmen, a holistic health geek with a passion for health, herbalism, natural remedies, as well as whole-food and plant-based lifestyles. After resolving various health issues I have struggled with for many years, I aim to inspire and help improve your health and longevity by sharing the tireless hours of research and valuable information I have discovered throughout my journey. Through the power of nutrition and lifestyle, with an evidence-based approach, I believe you can achieve your health and wellness goals.

If you enjoyed this book, I would love to hear how it has benefited you and invite you to leave a short review on Amazon - your valuable feed-back is always appreciated!

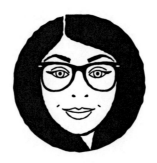

*You are invited to to join our **Free Book Club** mailing list. Sign up via our website to receive **special offers** and **free for a limited time** Health & Wellness eBooks!*

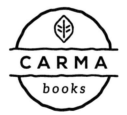

'A conscious approach to health & wellness'

carmabooks.com

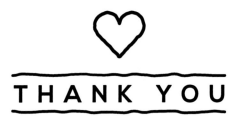

CPSIA information can be obtained
at www.ICGtesting.com
Printed in the USA
FSOW01n1105201216
28751FS